1

Introduction

Congratulations! By reading this book, it means you have decided to advance your career in the medical field by earning your Nursing Case Management certification. Before we get started, let's review some of the basic information. You are likely already familiar with this exam, the eligibility requirements, and so on, so we will keep it brief.

About the Exam

The Nursing Case Management exam is created and administered by the ANCC, or American Nurses Credentialing Center. The credential you will be awarded upon successful completion of the exam is referred to by the ANCC as "NE-BC". The actual exam is 175 questions (150 are scored, 25 are "pre-test" that are not scored) and you will have 3.5 hours to complete the entire test.

Eligibility Requirements

Per the ANCC, applicants for the NE-BC credential must:
- Hold a current, active RN license within a state or territory of the United States or the professional, legally recognized equivalent in another country.
- Hold a Bachelor's or higher degree in the field or nursing
- Have held a mid-level administrative or higher position such as a supervisor or director. Alternatively, have held a faculty position teaching graduate nursing students.
- Have completed 30 hours of continuing education in nursing administration within the last 3 years.

Applying for the Exam

You may apply by mail, or you can register online. In either case, you will need to find the ANCC website at www.nursecredentialing.org , find your certification under the "certification". Once you arrive at the introduction page for the Nursing Case Management page, you will see the instructions for completing the application online. If you want to do it by mail, you will need to download the application from online and then print and mail it in. If you have questions, you can always call their customer care team at 1-800-284-2378. There is a $395 fee to sit for this exam, or $270 if you are an ANCC member.

Preparing for the Exam

Obviously, you are already off to a great start by reading this book! However, there are of course additional resources you should use as well. When you visit the ANCC website to apply for the exam, be sure to look through the free resources available there. You can see an outline or "blueprint" of the exam, which is very helpful to familiarize yourself with the general concepts you'll see on the test. This won't provide any detail about the concepts, so it's not useful for in-depth studying like you will get in this book, but is certainly a good idea to be familiar with the outline of the exam. The more you know about and are familiar with the exam beforehand, the better you'll do. They also provide a few sample questions, so is a good place to get an initial assessment of your current knowledge if you like (we have a lot of practice questions in this book too of course). Finally, if you find yourself struggling with specific concepts, the ANCC has a list of references you can find to get very in-depth reviews. There are 25 different resources listed, so you obviously would never have time to read through everything, but is good to know about in case you need it later.

Nurse Executive Practice Test

1. What is another name for affirmative action?
    A. Employment equity
    B. Ethnic diversity
    C. Leveraging diversity
    D. Equal opportunity

2. Which nursing care delivery model proposes that a nurse hold 24-hour responsibility for a patient from admission through discharge?
    A. Team nursing
    B. Functional nursing
    C. Primary nursing
    D. Total patient care nursing

3. Medical waste disposal programs are primarily regulated on which level?
    A. Federal
    B. State
    C. Local
    D. Community

4. One approach to employee staffing that views people as assets is _____.
    A. Financial management
    B. Human capital management
    C. Staffing distribution
    D. Strategic alignment

5. Which area of basic financial management is usually under the direct control of the nurse executive?
    A. Revenue
    B. Staffing distribution
    C. Expense budget
    D. Alliance program

6. Which form of tangible property can be depreciated in the healthcare environment?
    A. Equipment
    B. Patents
    C. Computer software
    D. Patient care supplies

7. Which explains the difference between the staff mix and the staffing ratio?
   A. The staffing mix is a set numbers determined by legislation, particularly for intensive care units and emergency departments, whereas the staffing ratio is the ratio of various types of personnel to one another.
   B. The staffing mix is the determination of the number of personnel allocated per shift, whereas the staffing ratio is the ratio of various types of personnel to one another.
   C. The staffing mix is the ratio of various types of personnel to one another, whereas staffing ratios are set numbers determined by legislation, particularly for intensive care units and emergency departments.
   D. The terms are often used interchangeably.

8. Which type of costs remains constant for the healthcare facility regardless of fluctuations in activity levels such as fees and insurance premiums?
   A. Variable costs
   B. Fixed costs
   C. Fees
   D. Census

9. The purpose of the business plan is to:
   A. Show chief financial officers and elected board officials necessary information
   B. Help decision makers decide what to do and if this choice is right for the organization
   C. Provide economic values such as return on investment (ROI) and cost benefit analysis (CBA)
   D. All of the above

10. Which model of productivity is specific to nursing and measures the ratio of work output compared to work input?
    A. Systems framework
    B. Return on investment
    C. Cost benefit analysis
    D. Industrial model

11. All of the following are requirements for depreciation set by the IRS EXCEPT:
    A. The property must have a determinable useful life of one year or more.
    B. The taxpayer must use the property for business or in an income-producing manner.
    C. There can be no capital improvements from the property that is leased.
    D. The taxpayer must own the property.

12. When a nurse executive attempts to reduce the frequencies of injuries, accidents, and adverse events in the workplace, which concept is he/she using?
    A. Risk management
    B. Cost containment
    C. Reduction in staff
    D. Reduction in services

13. Which of the following is an approach to resource management where the payment applies to specified care coordination services by certain types of providers such as home healthcare?
    A. Fee for service
    B. Pay for performance
    C. Pay for coordination
    D. Bundled payments

14. The net value for a healthcare organization is often determined by:
    A. A cost-benefit analysis
    B. The quantified costs minus all the benefits
    C. The Resource-Based Relative Value Scale (RBRVS) system
    D. Payments for services

15. If a position requires 7-day coverage for a week, the FTE will be greater than 1.0 for that particular position such as in nursing care. A 7-day coverage where 8 hours each day must be covered would equal a _____ FTE.
    A. 1.0
    B. 1.4
    C. 1.8
    D. 2.0

16. If the total annual patient days equal 300, and the total number of beds is 200, what is the occupancy rate?
    A. 31%
    B. 40%
    C. 41%
    D. 50%

17. What value is determined by dividing total production hours by the number of patients?
    A. Full-time equivalent (FTE)
    B. Hours per patient day (HPPD)
    C. Average daily census
    D. Occupancy rate

18. What would the profit per inpatient discharge be if the inpatient revenue (net) was 3 million, the inpatient operating expenses were 1.5 million, and the total discharges were 50,000?
    A. $300
    B. $3,000
    C. $30,000
    D. $300,000

19. Under the Fair Labor Standards Act, which group is NOT considered exempt from overtime pay and minimum wage requirements?
    A. Professional nurses
    B. Administrative employees
    C. Apprentices
    D. Certified nursing assistants

20. How is the workload index determined?
    A. Multiply the number of production hours by the acuity index.
    B. Multiply the number of production hours by the workload units, and then divide that number by the acuity index.
    C. Multiply the acuity index by the workload units, and then divide by the number of production hours.
    D. None of the above

21. All of the following are true statements concerning a budget EXCEPT:
    A. A budget is a plan for coordinating financial goals for an organization.
    B. A budget provides necessary information to nurse executives and financial officers to develop actions to control results in the future.
    C. Nurse executives are expected to routinely analyze and monitor budget reports, usually monthly.
    D. The budget information provides a prospective history of financial activities.

22. Why should a nurse executive be familiar with historical trends regarding allocation when preparing a budget?
    A. Only under-correction of variance occurs when they are not considered.
    B. Both over- and under-correction of variance could occur when the trends are not considered.
    C. Neither over- nor under-correction of variance could occur when the trends are not considered.
    D. Historical trends regarding allocation are not important when preparing a budget.

23. Which type of budget involves renovation and equipment expenses necessary to meet long-term goals?
    A. Operating budget
    B. Capital budget
    C. Both A and B
    D. Neither A nor B

24. The Family Medical Leave Act applies only to certain employers. Which of the following would not be subject to FMLA rules and regulations?
    A. A private-sector employer with 30 employees in 20 or more workweeks in the current or preceding calendar year
    B. A state agency with 200 employees
    C. A federal agency with 20 employees
    D. A private elementary school with 100 employees

25. Under the Family Medical Leave Act, an eligible employee is someone who:
    • Works for a covered employer
    • Has worked for the employer for at least 6 months
    • Has at least 250 hours of service for the employer during that 6-month period
    • Works at a location where the employer has at least 30 employees

26. Eligible employees are entitled to 12 workweeks of leave in a one-year period under the Family Medical Leave Act, as long as certain conditions apply. Which of the following is NOT one of those conditions?
    • For the birth of a child and to care for the newborn during this timeframe
    • To care for a child, spouse, or parent with a serious health condition
    • To care for an adopted child or a child in newly placed foster care
    • For a minor health condition

27. Systems for monitoring the integrity of a healthcare facility for risk management purposes include all of the following EXCEPT:
    A. Committee meeting minutes
    B. Incident reports
    C. Audits
    D. Emails

28. Which of the following is NOT a reduction in force (RIF) cost-containment strategy?
    A. Outsourcing linen and laundry
    B. Using temporary staffing
    C. Scheduling fewer nurses
    D. Ordering cheaper supplies

29. Which of the following laws supports human capital management?
    A. Americans with Disabilities Act
    B. Federal Workforce Flexibility Act
    C. Family Medical Leave Act
    D. Civil Rights Act

30. Under the Americans with Disabilities Act, reasonable accommodations implies all of the following modifications EXCEPT:
    A. Modifications to the job application process that allow a qualified individual with a disability to be considered for a certain position
    B. Modifications that enable an employee with a disability to profit from the same privileges and benefits as those without disabilities
    C. Modifications to the work environment circumstances, or manner under which the position is held, that allow a qualified person with a disability to perform the necessary work functions
    D. Modifications that enable an employee with a disability to achieve certain privileges and benefits because of his/her disabilities

31. Under the Fair Labor Standards Act, a workweek is a regularly occurring period of _____ hours during seven consecutive 24-hour periods.
    A. 40
    B. 140
    C. 168
    D. 175

32. The Fair Labor Standards Act does NOT require and enforce which of the following?
    A. Employer record keeping
    B. Breaks and meal periods
    C. Minimum wage
    D. Overtime pay

33. Which agency or law requires that men and women performing equal work receive equal pay?
    A. FLSA Amendments of 1989
    B. Equal Pay Act of 1963
    C. Civil Rights Act of 1964
    D. Rehabilitation Act of 1973

34. Under the FLSA Child Labor Provisions law, the basic minimum age for employment is _____ years.
    A. 14
    B. 15
    C. 16
    D. 18

35. Which of the following employers are NOT subject to anti-discrimination laws under the Civil Rights Act of 1964, which is enforced by the Equal Employment Opportunity Commission?
    A. Those with 20 or fewer employees
    B. Paid volunteers
    C. Non-citizens of the U.S. who are employed overseas by U.S. employers
    D. Independent contractors

36. Which of the following issues would NOT qualify as an exception to the Civil Rights Act under the bonafide occupational qualification?
    A. Mobility problems
    B. Weight-bearing difficulties
    C. Trouble lifting
    D. Seasonal depression

37. Who is protected under the Age Discrimination in Employment Act of 1967?
    A. All American workers
    B. Individuals between the ages of 16 and 35
    C. Individuals between the ages of 40 and 70
    D. Individuals under the age of 16

38. Which corporate culture type is characterized by a "top-down" concept, with decisions made at the executive level and passed on to employees?
    A. Autocratic
    B. Bureaucratic
    C. Democratic
    D. Participative

39. All of the following statements are true concerning the Occupational Safety and Health Administration EXCEPT:
    A. OSHA covers any employer who operates or engages in a business that affects commerce.
    B. OSHA is authorized by the federal government to conduct a workplace inspection on any business.
    C. The U.S. Department of Labor governs OSHA.
    D. OSHA can conduct inspections in response to an employee complaint.

40. The Occupational Safety and Health Administration requires employers with _____ or more employees to keep records of work-related illnesses and injuries.
    A. 7
    B. 10
    C. 11
    D. 14

41. According to the current statistics reported by the Occupational Health and Safety Administration, at which rate has occupational and workplace injury and illness declined?
    A. 50%
    B. 57%
    C. 60%
    D. 67%

42. Which OSHA cooperative program is for employers with special interest and experience in job safety and health who also have a commitment to improving workplace safety?
    A. Alliance Program
    B. Voluntary Protection Program
    C. Strategic Partnership Program
    D. Challenge Program

43. Which sequence would represent an appropriate chain of command in the healthcare environment?
    A. Nurse Executive, RN Team Leader, Staff RN, CNA
    B. Nurse Executive, CNA, Staff RN, RN Team Leader
    C. CNA, Staff RN, RN Team Leader, Nurse Executive
    D. Nurse Executive, Director of Nursing, Chief Executive Officer, Hospital Board

44. Of the following people, who is NOT mandated by state law to report neglect and abuse of children and/or the elderly?
    A. Social workers
    B. Teachers
    C. Nurses
    D. Medical billers

45. Which of the following is NOT a cause of health disparities?
    A. Lack of education
    B. Poverty
    C. Environmental threats
    D. Occupation

46. Which is the most accurate description of lateral violence?
   A. Lateral violence is a form of harassment where nurses show aggressive or destructive behavior against each other or one group against a person or group.
   B. Lateral violence is a form of physical violence where one nurse assaults another.
   C. Lateral violence is a form of physical violence where a group of nurses assault one other person.
   D. Lateral violence is a form of harassment where the nurse executive shows aggressive or destructive behavior against his/her superiors.

47. Which type of network system involves direct communication in all directions without restriction?
   A. Centralized system
   B. Decentralized system
   C. Restricted system
   D. Unrestricted system

48. Which form of electronic data transfer is considered a first-level product that brings together data from other sources and delivers it electronically to the user?
   A. Computerized Medical Record System (CMRS)
   B. Electronic Medical Record (EMR)
   C. Electronic Patient Record (EPR)
   D. Automated Medical Record (AMR)

49. Which process of the regulation of the nursing profession is the process of granting permission to a person to practice?
   A. Certification
   B. Licensure
   C. Credentialing
   D. Registration

50. What is the purpose of the Joint Commission?
   A. To accredit acute care hospitals, critical access facilities, medical equipment services, home healthcare and hospice agencies, rehabilitation centers, physician practices, surgical centers, skilled nursing homes, and independent laboratories
   B. To set the standards for healthcare facilities and organizations
   C. Both A and B
   D. Neither A nor B

51. What is the difference between the Medicare and Medicaid programs?
    A. The Medicare program was an addendum to the Medicaid program.
    B. The Medicare program was aimed at the retirement age population and those with disabilities, whereas the Medicaid program was established for low-income children and their parents or guardians; those with developmental disabilities; and other low-income groups such as pregnant women, the elderly, and children.
    C. The Medicaid program was aimed at the retirement age population and those with disabilities, whereas the Medicare program was established for low-income children and their parents or guardians; those with developmental disabilities; and other low-income groups such as pregnant women, the elderly, and children.
    D. The Medicare program was created to replace the Medicaid program.

52. Which model was designed to provide direction for healthcare, allow multidisciplinary teams to communicate and collaborate, and define intended outcomes following the law of averages and evidence-based research?
    A. Shared governance model
    B. Traditional hierarchy
    C. Clinical pathways
    D. Career ladders

53. Which healthcare delivery model is a task-oriented method in which individual caregivers perform specific assigned tasks for all patients in a given unit or area?
    A. Case Method Nursing
    B. Team Nursing
    C. Functional Nursing
    D. Primary Nursing

54. What is the purpose of certification?
    A. To assure the public and concerned parties that an individual has mastered skills and knowledge in a certain area
    B. To designate when institutions or individuals have met the established standards set by an organization
    C. To accept the credentialing status of another credentialing body for specified purposes
    D. To show legal recognition of professional practice

55. Which of the following is NOT an aspect considered under the ANA Standards of Professional Performance?
    A. Ethics
    B. Research
    C. Education
    D. Diagnosis

56. Nurse Practice Acts (NPAs) are regulated on which level?
   A. Local
   B. State
   C. Federal
   D. None of the above

57. The four predictable stages of group development are:
   A. Team formation, team building, team structure, and team elimination
   B. Forming, storming, norming, and performing
   C. Starting, gathering, producing, evaluating
   D. Primary, secondary, tertiary, and quaternary

58. The Joint Commission's standard HR.01.04.01 requires hospitals and healthcare facilities to:
   A. Offer an orientation program that is 3 days long for temporary staff and 4-12 weeks long for long-term employees
   B. Offer a general facility orientation and a unit-specific orientation
   C. Offer a unit-specific orientation
   D. Offer a general facility orientation

59. Which is NOT true concerning competency validation during orientation?
   A. The Joint Commission standard HR.01.06.01 requires that staff competency be assessed and documented during orientation.
   B. Many worksites complete competency validation initially via a checklist.
   C. One competency validation tool is the Performance Based Development System (PBDS).
   D. Competency checklists are completely accurate concerning each person's perception of his/her abilities.

60. There is an accepted process that occurs in all areas of life and learning, which is defined as a purposeful, goal-directed, self-regulatory process that is context bound. What is this called?
   A. Cultural competence
   B. Critical thinking
   C. Leveraging diversity
   D. All three terms are interchangeable.

61. Conflict between two nurses who work in the same intensive care unit is called _____ conflict.
   A. Intrapersonal
   B. Interpersonal
   C. Intragroup
   D. Intergroup

62. A nurse executive knows that a person is upset based on his/her voice and facial expression. This is considered to be which element of emotional intelligence?
    A. Perceiving emotions
    B. Using emotions
    C. Managing emotions
    D. Understanding emotions

63. Which concept in healthcare focuses on the systematic and continuous actions that lead to a measurable improvement in healthcare services and in the health of patient populations?
    A. The Plan-Do-Study-Act (PDSA) cycle
    B. Quality improvement (QI)
    C. Communication systems
    D. None of the above

64. Which type of system interacts with the environment and internally?
    A. Closed system
    B. Open system
    C. Input system
    D. Output system

65. The nurse executive is discussing the use of a new electronic data transfer system during a staff meeting. One staff nurse asks a question, and the nurse leader explains a concept to that employee. When the staff nurse repeats back what she hears to the nurse executive, which type of communication has occurred?
    A. Active listening
    B. Reflective communication
    C. Two-way communication
    D. Interviewing

66. The preferred communication style in the healthcare environment is:
    A. Persuasive style
    B. Assertive style
    C. Passive style
    D. Both A and B
    E. Both B and C

67. What is a structured method for analyzing serious adverse events and identifying underlying problems that increase the likelihood of errors?
    A. Benchmarking
    B. Report cards
    C. Root cause analysis (RCA)
    D. Functional status

68. Suppose nursing researchers found that the misadministration of potassium chloride caused 100 preventable deaths in the U.S. healthcare system in 2013. What is this error considered to be?
    A. Nursing sensitive indicator
    B. Process indicator
    C. Structure indicator
    D. Sentinel event

69. Which type of healthcare improvement involves continually increasing quality to help healthcare facilities focus on vital interventions that have the greatest effect on health outcomes?
    A. Performance improvement (PI)
    B. Continuous quality improvement (CQI)
    C. Total quality management (TQM)
    D. Stakeholder satisfaction

70. Which type of indicators are part of the accreditation process of the Joint Commission that supplement and guide the standards-based survey process by providing a targeted basis for monitoring performance?
    A. Process indicators
    B. Structure indicators
    C. ORYX indicators
    D. Outcome indicators

71. What is the difference between a mission statement and a vision statement?
    A. A vision statement provides a general statement about the healthcare facility's purpose, and a mission statement describes the organization's goals and aspirations.
    B. A mission statement provides a general statement about the healthcare facility's purpose, and a vision statement describes the organization's goals and aspirations.
    C. The terms are used interchangeably.
    D. None of the above

72. A surgeon and a businessman open a surgical center. The surgeon will do the work, and the businessman will provide financing. Which type of organizational model is this?
    A. Vertical integration
    B. Horizontal integration
    C. Shared governance
    D. Joint venture

73. Which type of planning involves managing the business and determining what should be done before, during, and after an unexpected occurrence such as a tornado or earthquake?
    A. Strategic planning
    B. Contingency planning
    C. Program planning
    D. Healthy work environment

74. A nurse executive chooses not to attend a conference and instead uses the travel expense fund to buy his/her staff new uniforms. Which type of leader is this nurse executive?
    A. Charismatic leader
    B. Connective leader
    C. Servant leader
    D. Transactional leader

75. Concerning the behavior theory, which type of leader assumes that his/her subordinates can make their own decisions and that the staff need little direction?
    A. Autocratic
    B. Democratic
    C. Bureaucratic
    D. Permissive

76. Which change theory proposes that people maintain a state of equilibrium by balancing restraining and driving forces within any field?
    A. Maslow's Hierarchy of Needs Theory
    B. The Two-Factor Theory
    C. Lewin's Equilibrium Theory
    D. Rogers' Change Theory

77. Which type of planning provides smooth leadership transition for the organization to work with physicians to ensure high-quality standards and to groom new leaders?
    A. Contingency planning
    B. Financial planning
    C. Strategic planning
    D. Succession planning

78. During a nursing research project, you and your colleagues investigate a group of patients with community-acquired pneumonia. Which type of research is this?
    A. Applied research
    B. Case study research
    C. Descriptive research
    D. Experimental research

79. You are doing an observational research study regarding emergency and trauma nursing. This research is conducted in a natural setting, which is the emergency department. Which type of research is this?
    A. Field research
    B. Historical research
    C. Laboratory research
    D. Longitudinal research

80. Which group or agency ensures that research participants are protected from unethical and unscrupulous practices and researchers?
    A. Food and Drug Administration
    B. National Advisory Council for Nursing Research (NACNR)
    C. Institutional Review Board (IRB)
    D. Nursing Research Council

81. In a research report, you read that patients were listed by socioeconomic status. You understand that this data is ordered, but differences cannot be determined. Which type of data is this?
    A. Nominal
    B. Ordinal
    C. Interval
    D. Qualitative

82. Which statement concerning instrument values is true?
    A. An instrument can be valid without being reliable.
    B. An instrument can be reliable without being valid.
    C. An instrument cannot be valid if it is reliable.
    D. An instrument cannot be reliable if it is valid.

83. There are several dimensions of strategic innovation, which are intertwined to produce growth-oriented results. Which dimension helps understand emerging trends?
    A. Strategic alignment
    B. Industry foresight
    C. Patient insight
    D. Organizational readiness

84. Which phase of the strategic innovation approach is characterized as open-ended and exploratory?
    A. Emergence phase
    B. Convergence phase
    C. Divergence phase
    D. None of the above

85. Equal employment laws involve various aspects of discrimination due to all of the following EXCEPT:
    A. Color/race/ethnicity
    B. Religion
    C. Age
    D. Sex
    E. Socioeconomic status

86. Considering the following, which benefit is not covered under the Workers' Compensation law?
    A. Medical coverage
    B. Costs of rehabilitation
    C. A percentage of wages or salary
    D. Bonus compensation for minor injury

87. An agreement negotiated between an employer and a labor union that sets forth the terms of employment for labor union workers is called:
    A. Grievance
    B. Arbitration
    C. Collective bargaining
    D. Contract

88. Why should a nurse executive demand a contract with the healthcare facility where she is employed?
    A. A contract will protect the nursing professional financially and secure job status.
    B. Contracts define the responsibilities and liabilities of employees, contractors, and/or other service providers.
    C. A contract will help the nurse secure a position that can otherwise be eliminated or restructured in the healthcare environment.
    D. All of the above

89. Which of the following is a way of thinking that allows the nurse executive to come up with original ideas and creative solutions to various problems?
    A. Critical thinking
    B. Lateral thinking
    C. Vertical thinking
    D. Logical thinking

90. A surgical team is reimbursed with one large sum for all services provided during a procedure. This is an example of _____.
    A. Fee for service payment
    B. Pay for performance
    C. Pay for coordination
    D. Bundled payment

91. Hours per patient day (HPPD) are calculated by:
    A. Dividing total production hours by the number of patient days
    B. Dividing number of patient days by the total production hours
    C. Dividing the total annual patient days by 365
    D. Dividing the number of days in one year by the total annual patient days

92. What is the purpose of amortization?
    A. It allows for easy calculation of profit or loss.
    B. It is an assignment of costs to a capital item for its lifetime, so there can be development of a replacement strategy.
    C. It measures inpatient volume based on the number of occupied beds or number of patients.
    D. All of the above

93. Which of the following statements concerning Healthy People 2020 is NOT true?
    A. Healthy People creates benchmarks to measure the impact of preventive activities.
    B. Healthy People reflects input from only one prestigious organization.
    C. Healthy People is a 10-year agenda for improving the nation's health.
    D. Healthy People aims to increase public awareness of the determinants of disability and disease.

94. Of the following health disparities, which were found in the recent report by the Agency for Healthcare Research and Quality?
    A. Poor people had worse access to care than high-income people.
    B. Blacks, American Indians, Asians, Native Alaskans, and Hispanics received worse care than Whites.
    C. In 2002, 24% of Americans had difficulties accessing healthcare, and by 2009, this had increased to 26%.
    D. All of the above

95. What does the Affordable Care Act of 2010 contain?
    A. It calls for the creation of the Patient-Centered Outcomes Research Institute, which studies comparative effectiveness research.
    B. It allows the FDA to approve generic drugs.
    C. It has programs that increase incentives to provide collaborative and quality healthcare.
    D. All of the above

96. A nurse executive discovers that the physicians he/she works for are engaged in a gross waste of funds and abuse of authority. Which law would protect this nurse who plans to report the misconduct?
    A. Health Insurance Portability and Accountability Act
    B. Whistleblower Protection Act
    C. Fair Labor Standards Act
    D. Civil Rights Act

97. Which organization developed HCAHPS?
   A. Centers for Medicare and Medicaid Services (CMS)
   B. Agency for Healthcare Research and Quality (AHRQ)
   C. Both A and B
   D. Neither A nor B

98. Which type of network involves many local networks with connections that are affected by specialized networking software?
   A. Decentralized system
   B. Centralized system
   C. Local area network
   D. Wide area network

99. Which type of legislation allows a nurse licensed in one state to practice in other states without having to apply for a second license?
   A. Nurse compact legislation
   B. Federal legislation
   C. State legislation
   D. Recognition legislation

Test Your Knowledge—Answers

1. **A.**

   Affirmative action (also called employment equity) promotes equal opportunity and ethnic diversity in the workplace, in public contracting, in education, and in health programs. Ethnic diversity is the quality of diverse and different ethnic groups or persons, as opposed to a monoculture. Leveraging diversity fosters an inclusive workplace where diversity and individual differences are valued and leveraged to achieve the vision and mission of the organization. Equal opportunity is fairness of various opportunities (Rundio & Wilson, 2010).

2. **C.**

   The framework of how nursing care is delivered is called a nursing care delivery model. The four classic models are: team, functional, primary, and total patient care. In team nursing, a team leader (RN) manages the care for a small group of patients. In functional nursing, each nurse performs specific assigned tasks for all patients in a given area. In primary nursing, the RN performs advanced nursing function for a group of patients for a 24-hour time period and from admission through discharge. With total patient care nursing, the RN is responsible for all indirect and direct patient care functions, and he or she communicates needs, changes, and request for assistance with a charge nurse or team leader (Robinson, 2010).

3. **A.**

   The Environmental Protection Agency (EPA) implements laws to protect human health and the environment on the federal level, and this organization provides guidelines for the states. Biomedical waste programs and rules regarding disposal are primarily regulated on the state level.

4. **B.**

   Human capital management (HCM) is an approach to employee staffing that views people as assets (human capital). Financial management is an approach to allocation of resources. Staffing distribution is the determination of the number of personnel allocated per shift. Many healthcare facilities require 45% for day shift, 35% for evening shift, and 20% for night shift. Strategic alignment is part of a human capital management, where goals, mission and organizational objectives are all considered (Rundio & Wilson, 2010).

5. **B.**

   Revenue is the total amount of income anticipated during a specified period of time, and it is not usually under the direct control of nurse executives. Rather, a certain percentage of anticipated or actual revenue is allocated to the numerous cost centers. Staffing distribution is the determination of the number of personnel allocated per shift and nurse executives are usually responsible for this. The expense budget contains both salary and non-salary items, and most nurse executives are responsible for managing expenditures within an assigned cost center, which implies outflow of cash and/or resources, but not the entire budget. The Alliance Program works in conjunction with several other organizations that are involved with workplace health and safety not budgeting (Rundio & Wilson, 2010).

6. **A.**
Depreciation is an income tax deduction that is an annual allowance for the wear-and-tear or deterioration of the property. It allows a taxpayer to recover the costs or other aspects of specific property. Many types of tangible property can be depreciated, such as machinery, equipment, buildings, furniture, and vehicles. Intangible property is also depreciable, including copyrights, patents, and computer software. Patient care supplies are not considered tangible or intangible property (Internal Revenue Service, 2012).

7. **D.**
Staffing distribution is the determination of the number of personnel allocated per shift. The staffing mix (also called the staffing ratio) is the ratio of various types of personnel to one another. The staff mix may be more or less weighted toward the use of RNs, depending on the philosophy of the facility. Staffing ratios are often determined by legislation, particularly for intensive care units and emergency departments (Rundio & Wilson, 2010).

8. **B.**
Some healthcare facilities require the nurse manager to handle a profit center, which relates to an inflow of cash. Costs are either fixed or variable: fixed costs, which remain constant for the facility regardless of fluctuations inactivity levels, such as fees and insurance premiums, and variable costs, which fluctuate in response to either an external or internal influence, such as patient acuity, census, staff mix, and product cost (Rundio & Wilson, 2010).

9. **D.**
A business plan uses economic justification to show chief financial officers and elected board officials the necessary information. This plan helps decision makers decide what to do and if the choice is right for the organization. The ROI is a calculation of the most tangible financial gains or benefits that are expected from a given project compared to the costs for implementing a program or solution. The cost benefit analysis (CBA) is similar to the ROI, but more comprehensive in that it attempts to quantify both tangible and intangible (soft) benefits and costs (Federal Geographic Data Committee. 2009).

10. **D.**
There are two models of productivity that are specific to nursing: the *industrial model* and the *systems framework*. The industrial model measure the ratio of work output to work input and is considered representative of efficiency. The systems framework involves both efficiency and efficacy, with efficiency including nursing

output and efficacy including quality and appropriateness (Rundio & Wilson, 2010).

11. **C.**

The requirements for depreciation set by the Internal Revenue Service (2012) include: (1) the property must have a determinable useful life of one year or more; (2) the taxpayer must own the property; (3) the taxpayer can depreciate any capital improvements from property that is leased; and (4) the taxpayer must use the property for business or in an income-producing aspect. If the property is used for personal purposes as well as business, the taxpayer can only deduct depreciation based only on the business use.

12. **A.**

Risk management is significant in the healthcare arena, especially with commitments and mandates related to disclosure of adverse events. Risk management is a problem-focused approach to reduce the frequency and severity of injuries, accidents, and adverse events. Cost containment is an approach to managing finances that employs such strategies as risk management, reduction in staff, and reduction in services (Rundio & Wilson, 2010).

13. **C.**

The pay per coordination (PPC) benefits are linked with the concept of paying for care coordination, which involves support services or other work that is not available under a fee for service model. Fee for service reimbursement is the standard payment option that relates to one payment for one service. Under a pay for performance (PFP) approach, the healthcare insurer or other payer compensates healthcare facilities and physicians based on performance. With bundled payments, a single, bundled payment covers the services delivered by two or more providers during a single care episode over a certain period of time (American Medical Association, 2013).

14. **A.**

The cost-benefit analysis is the exercise of evaluating a planned action by determining what net value for the organization. A CBA finds and quantifies all of the positive factors (benefits) and identifies, quantifies, and subtracts all the negative factors (costs). The difference between the two values indicates whether a planned action is profitable. The Resource-Based Relative Value Scale System (RBRVS) establishes a standardized payment schedule based on resource-based scale. With the RBRVS, payments are calculated by multiplying the costs of a service by a monetary amount determined by the Centers for Medicare and Medicaid Services (Internal Revenue Service, 2012).

15. **B.**

Total hours is 56 (7 multiplied by 8). FTE is total hours divided by 40, which is the workweek. This value is 1.4 (Rundio & Wilson, 2010).

16. **C.**

The occupancy rate is the total annual patient days divided by the number of beds multiplied by 365, then that value multiplied by 100. This value measures inpatient volume as a percentage of the number of occupied beds. The higher the occupancy rate, the better profitability, unless it is exceedingly high. To raise this rate, healthcare facilities can increase admissions, decrease the number of beds, or increase the length of patient stay. This measure is often called occupancy.

$$\text{Occupancy Rate} = \frac{\text{Total Annual Patient Days} * 100}{\text{Number of Beds} * 365}$$

17. **B.**

The hours of nursing care that must be provided per patient per day is considered the hours per patient day (HPPD). This value is determined by dividing total production hours by the number of patients. Full-time equivalent is the number of hours of work for which a full-time employee is scheduled for a work week. The average daily census is the total annual patient days divided by 365. The occupancy rate is the total annual patient days divided by the number of beds multiplied by 365, then that value multiplied by 100 (American College of Healthcare Executives, 2013).

18. **A.**

The profit per inpatient discharge is the inpatient revenue (net) minus the inpatient operating expenses divided by total discharges. This measures the amount of profit that is earned on inpatient discharge. Low values are negative numbers, which can be traced either to low inpatient reimbursement or high inpatient costs or both. The lack of inpatient profitability can lead to serious financial difficulties (American College of Healthcare Executives, 2013).

19. **D.**

Unless exempted, employees covered by the FLSA must receive overtime pay for all hours worked in excess of 40 hours in a work week at a minimum rate of time and one-half of their regular rate of pay. Certain employees are considered "white-collar" exemptions, such as executive, professional, and administrative employees. Others who are subject to exemptions include apprentices, students and those individuals subject to child labor regulations (U.S. Department of Labor, 2013).

20. **C.**

The workload index is weighted statistics that reflect the acuity level of patients, census, and production hours. This index often functions as a baseline for productivity improvement. To get the workload index, you multiply the acuity index by the workload units and then divide by the number of production hours (Rundio & Wilson, 2010).

$$\frac{\text{Acuity Index} \times \text{Workload Units}}{\text{Production Hours}}$$

21. **D.**

The budget information provides a retrospective (not prospective) history of financial activities. All the other statements are correct.

22. **B.**

The budget information provides three things: a history of financial activities that is retrospective; the status of each unit or department; and the anticipated revenue for the upcoming year. Nurse executives need to be familiar with these trends, as well as the trending methodology used in the organization. Over- or under-correction of variance could occur when the trends are not considered, leading to difficulties in the future months (Rundio & Wilson, 2010).

23. **B.**

The *capital budget* involves renovation and equipment expenses necessary to meet long-term goals. The *operating budget* (also called an annual budget) is based on anticipated expenses and revenues for the *fiscal year*, which is 12 months that do not always occur in the order of the calendar year (Rundio & Wilson, 2010).

24. **A.**

Covered employers include: private-sector employer with 50 (not 30) or more employees in 20 or more work weeks in the current or preceding calendar year, including a successor or joint employer in interest to a covered employer; public agency, including local, state, or federal agencies regardless of the number of employees; public or private elementary or secondary schools, regardless of the number of employees (Rundio & Wilson, 2010).

25. **A.**

An eligible employee is someone who:
- Works for a covered employer
- Has worked for the employer for at least 12 months (not 6 months)
- Has at least 1,250 hours (not 250) of service for the employer during that 12 month period (not 6 months)
- Works at a location where the employer has at least 50 employees (not 30)

(Rundio & Wilson, 2010)

26. **D.**

Eligible employees are entitled to 12 work weeks of leave in a year period under the FMLA: for the birth of a child and to care for the newborn during this timeframe; to care for a child, spouse, or parent who has a serious health condition; to care for an adopted child or a child in newly placed foster care; for a serious health condition that makes the employee unable to work (not a minor health condition; and for any qualifying exigency arising from the fact that the employee's spouse, son, daughter, or parent is a covered military member on "covered active duty" (U.S. Department of Labor, 2013a).

27. **D.**

One of the main components of a risk management program is review of monitoring systems regarding their integrity, including questionnaires, incident reports, meeting minutes of various committees, audits, and oral complaints (Rundio & Wilson, 2010).

28. **D.**

Outsourcing is one approach to cost containment, such as housekeeping, linen and laundry, food services, payroll, transcription, and data processing. Temporary agencies can supply core staff to satisfy seasonal requirements when necessary. Cost savings achieved through RIFs may not always be sustained, as hidden cost could outweigh the anticipated savings (Rundio & Wilson, 2010).

29. **B.**

The Federal Workforce Flexibility Act of 2004 added many strategies that support human capital management (U.S. Office of Personnel Management, 2013). The Americans with Disabilities Act ensures that qualified individuals with disabilities enjoy the same employment opportunities as those who do not have any physical or mental disability (U.S. Department of Justice, 2013). The Family and Medical Leave Act (FMLA) entitles eligible employees of certain covered employers to take unpaid, job-protected leave for specified medical and family reasons with continuation of group health insurance coverage (U.S. Department of Labor, 2013a). Under the Civil Rights Act, employers cannot discriminate against an employee based on factors not related to job qualifications, such as age, sexual preference, religion, race, sex, or national origin (U.S. Equal Employment Opportunity Commission, 2013b).

30. **D.**

According to the EEOC, reasonable accommodation means modifications that enable an employee with a disability to achieve the same privileges and benefits as those who do not have disabilities. It does not guarantee privileges or benefits because of the disability (U.S. Department of Justice, 2013).

31. **C.**

The FLSA sets a minimum wage below which no covered employee may be legally employed, but the law sets a maximum number of hours in a workweek. A workweek is a regularly reoccurring period of 168 hours during seven consecutive 24-hour periods. Hours worked includes all the time an employee must remain on duty on the employer's premises or at the designated worksite and all the time the employee must work for the employer (U.S. Department of Labor, 2013).

32. **B.**

The FLSA does not require that employers give breaks or meal periods to workers, but some states implement these requirements (U.S. Department of Labor, 2013). The other choices (A, C, and D) are all things that the FLSA does require.

33. **B.**

The Equal Pay Act (EPA) of 1964 prohibits discrimination based on gender regarding compensation for work services (Rundio & Wilson, 2010). The U.S. Labor Department's Wage and Hour Division implemented amendments to the Fair Labor Standards Act (FLSA) in 1989 requiring employees lacking basic skills to receive additional remedial training in addition to their 40-hour work week. Under the Civil Rights Act of 1964, employers cannot discriminate against an employee based on factors not related to job qualifications, such as age, sexual preference, religion, race, sex, or national origin (U.S. Equal Employment Opportunity Commission, 2013b). The Rehabilitation Act of 1973 ensures that qualified individuals with handicaps are not excluded from participation in various programs and activities, or denied benefits from the employer (U.S. Equal Opportunity Commission, 2013d).

34. **C.**

The FLSA Child Labor Provisions law states that the basic minimum age for employment, which is 16 years. However, employment of 14 and 15 year old youths is allowed for certain occupations and under specific guidelines (Rundio & Wilson, 2010).

35. **D.**

Employers who are not subject to anti-discrimination laws include:
- those with 15 or fewer employees (not 20 – choice A)
- joint labor-management committees that control job training programs
- labor organizations
- independent contractors
- unpaid volunteers (not paid volunteers – choice B)
- non-citizens employed overseas by U.S. employers (not U.S. citizens – choice C)

(U.S. Equal Employment Opportunity Commission, 2013b)

36. **D.**

This Civil Rights Act corrects injustices and bias through affirmative action and other mechanisms. This permits employers from "screening out" certain people who are qualified for employment. One exception to this act is bonafide occupational qualification (BFOQ), where certain challenges are more difficult or unattainable due to age. BFOQs include weight-bearing and mobility issues, such as stairs, lifting, and other physical challenges (U.S. Equal Employment Opportunity Commission, 2013b).

37. **C.**

Congress enacted the Age Discrimination in Employment Act (ADEA) in 1967 to prevent arbitrary age discrimination in regards to employment, assists employers and workers discover ways to solve problems arising from the impact of age on employment. Individuals protect by ADEA include those who are between the ages of 40 and 70 years (U.S. Equal Opportunity Commission, 2013c).

38. **A.**

With the autocratic culture, managers and supervisors must enforce the decisions and help staff accept various decisions and changes. Techniques of an autocratic organization include coercion, direction of actions, and threats of punishment. In many organizations, the success of the facility depends on autocracy. A bureaucratic culture relies on rules, regulations, procedures, and policies. A participative culture is characterized by openness to recommendations and suggestions from all levels within the facility for the purpose of decision making. There is no democratic culture considered (Rundio & Wilson, 2010).

39. **B.**

OSHA is authorized to conduct workplace inspection on each business that is covered by the OSHA act. The U.S. Department of Labor is the federal department that governs OSHA. This organization allows OSHA to conduct an inspection at the request of the employer or in response to an employee complaint (Rundio & Wilson, 2010). The other choices (A, C, and D) are all correct statements.

40. **C.**

OSHA requires employers to keep certain records. OSHA supplies certain forms to employers available through the Internet and OSHA website. Employers with 11 or more employees must keep records of work-related illnesses and injuries (OSHA, 2013d).

41. **D.**

According to current statistics reported by OSHA, workplace injuries and illness rates have declined by 67 percent and occupational deaths have decreased by more than 65 percent (OSHA, 2013c).

42. **C.**

The Voluntary Protection Program (VPP) is used to document lost workday cases. The Alliance Program works in conjunction with several other organizations that are involved with workplace health and safety. The Challenge Program provides interested employers and employees the opportunity to gain assistance in improving their health and safety management systems (OSHA, 2013e).

43. **A.**

The *chain of command* refers to the line of command that exists from the top to the bottom of an organization. The chain of command allows for a smooth exchange of information. Each subsequent layer of the chain of command must report to the one immediately above it (Rundio & Wilson, 2010).

44. **D.**

Approximately 48 states and the District of Columbia designate professions whose members are mandated by law to notify authorities of child and elder maltreatment. These people include:

- Social workers
- Physicians, nurses, and other healthcare workers
- Medical examiners and coroners
- Teachers, principals, and other school personnel
- Child care providers and daycare workers
- Counselors, therapists, and other mental health professionals
- Law enforcement officers

(Child Information Gateway, 2012)

45. **D.**

The causes of health disparities include poverty, inadequate access to health care, lack of education, individual and behavioral factors, and environmental threats (Centers for Disease Control and Prevention, 2013b).

46. **A.**

Lateral violence results in damage to someone's confidence, self-esteem, or dignity. Lateral violence can consist of intentional and unintentional acts meant to intimidate, harm, or humiliate a person or group of people. This form of *harassment* puts patients and other workers at risk for poor outcomes (Rundio & Wilson, 2010).

47. **B.**

Networks allow entities to communicate, and they are a means to consolidate power, a mode for market sharing, or a way to enhance fiscal solvency through collective purchasing power. In a *decentralized system*, direct communication occurs in all directions and without restriction. With a *centralized system*, communication requires that input and output is controlled through a central point. Finally, a *restricted system* places international barriers between organizations and groups. There is no unrestricted system (Rudio & Wilson, 2010).

48. **D.**

The Computerized Medical Record System (CMRS) is a second-level product, where paper-based items are now are available electronically via scanning. The Electronic Medical Record (EMR) is a third-level product that provides capability for electronic information and data entry, data integrity, auditing, and electronic signature. The Electronic Patient Record (EPR) is a fourth-level product that brings together patient information from more than one organization or healthcare facility. The Electronic Health Record (EHR) is a fifth-level product that provides the user with information about the patient from multiple sources, including data not pertaining to his or her medical problem or health condition (Rundio & Wilson, 2010).

49. **B.**

Licensure is the mandatory process of granting permission to a person to practice in a given profession. The purpose of licensure is to protect the public from unlicensed or untrained persons. *Certification* gives recognition to nurse who meet certain requirements, generally for a particular field or clinical specialty, but it does not include a legal scope of nursing practice. *Credentialing* is the process of awarding special recognition to those who meet certain requirements. *Registration* involves board control the nursing licensure process and "register" nurses to practice under the rules and regulations of that governing body (Rundio & Wilson, 2010).

50. **C.**

The Joint Commission on the Accreditation of Hospitals (JCAH) was established in 1951, and it sets the standards for approximately 16,000 healthcare facilities in America. Joint Commission also accredits acute care hospitals, critical access facilities, medical equipment services, home healthcare and hospice agencies, rehabilitation centers, physician practices, surgical centers, skilled nursing homes, and independent laboratories (Rundio & Wilson, 2010).

51. **B.**

The Medicare program was aimed at the retirement age population and those with disabilities, whereas the Medicaid program was established for low income children and their parents or guardians, those with developmental disabilities, and other low income groups, such as pregnant women, the elderly, and children.

52. **C.**

The *shared governance model* allows staff nurses to be part of the decision-making process about the healthcare facility or their unit or service. In the *traditional hierarchy*, the staff nurses report to a charge nurse, who reports to a nurse manager, who reports to a nurse executive, and on up the chain of command. *Clinical advancement programs* (also called *career ladders* or *clinical ladders*) foster recognition of professional and expert nurses and offer a career pathway that will allow them to continue providing direct care to patients (Rundio & Wilson, 2010).

53. **C.**

The *functional nursing* care delivery system is a task-oriented method in which individual caregivers are not assigned to patients. The *case method nursing* care approach is often practiced in intensive care settings or in home healthcare settings. In addition to the nursing process, the RN is responsible for all indirect and direct patient care functions, and he or she communicates needs, changes, and request for assistance with a charge nurse or team leader. With *team nursing*, patients are assigned to a team of nurses, therapists, dieticians, and assistants. *Primary nursing* is a patient care system where a primary nurse is responsible for planning the patient's care and delegating tasks when he or she is not present (Robinson, 2010).

54. **A.**

Credentialing is a termed used to describe the processes used for program designation when institutions or individuals have met the established standards set by an organization (American Nurses Association, 1979). *Recognition* is the process where an association, organization, or agency accepts the credentialing status of another credentialing body for specified purposes (American Nurses Association, 2004). *Licensure* is the process of legal recognition of professional practice (Rundio & Wilson, 2010).

55. **D.**

The American Nurses Association (ANA) has developed standards for nursing practice and the scope of practice. The *standards of nursing care* are guidelines for practice, which are general to any specialty or setting, and they include the broad categories of assessment, diagnosis, outcome identification, planning, implementation, and evaluation. The *standards of professional performance* address the nursing role with regard to ethics, research, education, collegiality, and resource utilization (Robinson, 2010).

56. **B.**

The U.S. Nurse Practice Acts are legislations that guide and govern nursing practice. All states have enacted a Nurse Practice Act (NPA), and each state NPA is enforced by the state's legislature (National Council of State Boards of Nursing, 2013).

57. **B.**

There are four predictable stages of *group development*: *forming*, where individuals come together and form a group; *storming*, where the group proceeds through the maturation process and identifies a leader; *norming*, where the rules of working as a group are made explicit and roles and relationships are clarified; and *performing*, where the group does most of the work and focuses energies on achieving goals (Rundio & Wilson, 2010).

58. **B.**

The Joint Commission (2009) requires hospitals and healthcare facilities to orient staff with both relevant hospital-wide and unit-specific programs that both focus on policies and procedures. An orientation program typically ranges from three days for temporary staff to four to twelve weeks for long-term employees. This length of orientation is set by the organization and should be clearly communicated to the employee (Galvak, 2007).

59. **D.**

The Joint Commission standard HR.01.06.01 requires that staff *competency* be assessed and documented during orientation. One competency validation tool is the Performance Based Development System (PBDS). Many worksites accomplish *competency validation* initially via a check list. These check lists are NOT completely accurate, as each person's perception of his or her abilities varies (The Joint Commission, 2009).

60. **B.**

The nurse must have the ability to think critically, as well as use sound clinical judgment. *Critical thinking* is not a class that is taught, nor is it a body of knowledge learned. *Cultural competence* is defined as the ability to interact well people of different ethnicities and cultures with a focus on personal awareness of one's own attitude toward couture. *Leveraging diversity* is the ability of a facility to become culturally competent and value diversity from a business and personal perspective (Osborn, Wraa, & Watson, 2010; Rundio & Wilson, 2010).

61. **C.**

With intrapersonal conflict, the conflict is within oneself. With interpersonal conflict, the conflict is between the self and another person. The conflict is considered intragroup when it is among members of a group. Intergroup conflict is among members of two or more groups (Rundio & Wilson, 2010).

62. **A.**

The Ability-Based Model for Emotional Intelligence provides a framework for the concept of emotional intelligence. Perceiving emotions is the ability to detect emotions in voices, faces, and cultural artifacts, as well as the ability to identify one's own emotional state. Using emotions is the ability to use emotions to facilitate cognitive activities such as thinking and problem solving. Managing emotions is the ability to regulate emotions in others and ourselves. Understanding emotions is the ability to understand emotional language (Rundio & Wilson, 2010).

63. **B.**

Quality in healthcare is a direct correlation between the level of improved health services and the desired outcomes of patients and/or patient populations. The Plan-Do-Study-Act (PDSA) cycle is part of the Institute for Healthcare Improvement Model. This is a simple tool used to accelerate quality improvement. Communication systems are formal and informal structures used to support the communication needs within an organization (Coiera, 2006; U.S. Department of Health and Human Services, 2013d).

64. **B.**

Systems are either closed or open. *Closed systems* occur only in physical sciences, such as the circulatory system. *Open systems* interact with the environment and internally. The parts of this system are input, throughput, and output (Rundio & Wilson, 2010).

65. **A.**

With active listening, the listener repeats back what they hear to the speaker to confirm understanding between both parties (Wikipedia, 2013a). Reflective communication involves seeking to understand the speaker's idea, the offer the idea back to the speaker in an attempt to reconstruct the idea and relay understanding (Wikipedia, 2013b).Two-way communication is a form of transmission in which both parties transmit information, such as chatrooms, instant messaging, telephone conversations, and in-person discussions (Wikipedia, 2013c). An interview is a conversation between two or more people, which is done in medial reporting, in qualitative research, in employee statements, and to receive the facts.

66. **D.**

One preferred style of communication is the persuasive style. This style encourages others to view ideas as beneficial to their needs, displays authority to build trust, and reassures staff by creating an emotive and empathetic connection. The assertive communication style involves standing up for personal rights and expressing feelings, beliefs, and thoughts in an honest, direct, and appropriate way which does not violate another individual's rights. It is also a preferred communication style. The passive style involves violating your own rights by failing to express your feelings, beliefs, and thoughts and allowing others to violate your rights, and it is not preferred (Richerson & Watson, 2010).

67. **C.**

The goal of RCA is to identify both active and latent errors, those that are hidden. *Benchmarking* is a technique that identifies top quality as a means of comparing one's practice or healthcare facility with those who are judged objectively to be the standard or pacesetter of a certain category. *Report cards* are issued by accrediting bodies, such as payers or The Joint Commission. Functional areas within an organization must accurately perform the work for which they are accountable so that the organization can achieve goals and surpass competitors. The *functional status* of an organization involves areas that are interdependent (Rundio & Wilson, 2010).

68. **D.**

Sentinel events are unexpected occurrences that have the potential to result in or actually cause death or injury (Richerson & Watson, 2010). *Nursing sensitive indicators* are associated with the process, structure, and outcomes of nursing care. *Process indicators* measure aspects of nursing care, such as assessment and intervention. *Structure indicators* measure the supply of nursing staff, the staff member's skill level, and the education and certification of nursing staff. *Outcome indicators* are specific to patient outcomes or quality of nursing care, such as intravenous infiltrations or falls (American Nurses Association, 2013b).

69. **B.**

Continuous quality improvement (CQI) is the process of continually increasing quality. *Performance improvement* (PI) activities are those that involve the quality structure of most healthcare facilities and medical organizations. *Total quality management* (TQM) is the process where everyone employed by the healthcare facility is committed to continuous improvement. There are many *stakeholders* who have a vested interest in a healthcare organization, such as the patient and family, the staff, the physicians, and the payers. Stakeholder satisfaction is when these persons approve of the healthcare organization (Rundio & Wilson, 2010).

70. **C.**

ORYX indicators are part of the accreditation process that integrates outcomes and other performance improvement data. ORYX measurement requirements support Joint Commission accredited healthcare facilities in their quality improvement efforts (The Joint Commission, 2013a). *Process indicators* measure aspects of nursing care, such as assessment and intervention. *Structure indicators* measure the supply of nursing staff, the staff member's skill level, and the education and certification of nursing staff.

Outcome indicators are specific to patient outcomes or quality of nursing care, such as intravenous infiltrations or falls (American Nurses Association, 2013b).

71. **B.**

These statements are meant to motivate and inspire those who are affiliated with the healthcare facility, and they are future-oriented and address what the facility plans to do give its resources. Most of these involve statements about the staff and administration (Rundio & Wilson, 2010).

72. **D.**

Organizations are structured in several ways. In a joint venture, one partner provides a service, and the other partner provides financing. With the vertical integration model, there is different but complementary services available to all parties, such as the affiliation with a HMO and a hospital. In horizontal integration, services are shared across two or more organizations, such as the provision of oncology services by one and the provision of orthopedic services by the other. Shared governance fosters ownership of work that is done by involvement of workers in decisions about staffing, performance, structure, and resource allocation (Rundio & Wilson, 2010).

73. **B.**

The *contingency plan* is the way the healthcare facility operates on a day-to-day basis, and it includes adverse events (Rundio & Wilson, 2010). *Strategic planning* is the development of an organizational strategy that will provide a long-term road map for a healthcare facility (Varkey & Bennet, 2010). *Program planning* is the organization's capacity to successfully execute a plan or service. With this process, the programs must match the organization's philosophy and beliefs to create a profit for the healthcare facility (Rundio & Wilson, 2010). A healthy work environment is a culture of collaborative practice, accountability, and communication (Sherman & Pross, 2010).

74. **C.**

Servant leaders put other people and their needs before their own and choose to lead by serving the interests of others. Charismatic leaders have the ability to engage others with the power of their personalities, and they inspire emotional connection and use charisma to advance revolutionary ideas. Connective leaders draw on their ability to bring others together to facilitate change. Transactional leaders associate with the principles of social-exchange theory, which implies that social, psychological, and political benefits exist in all relationships, such as that of the leader and follower (Rundio & Wilson, 2010).

75. **D.**

Permissive leaders have a lot of faith in their subordinates, assuming they can make good decisions and need little direction. Autocratic leaders attempt to change the behavior of subordinates through external control by coercion, punishment, authority, and power. Democratic leaders focus on changing subordinates through participation, involvement in goal setting, and collaboration. Bureaucratic leaders rely on the healthcare facility policies and rules to control and influence subordinates (Rundio & Wilson, 2010).

76. **C.**

Lewin proposed that people maintain a state of equilibrium, and for this to occur, there must be a disruption of balance. To lessen the power of restraining forces, one must either increase the force or decrease the power of the force. With *Maslow's Hierarchy of Needs Theory*, there are five basic needs that are common to all people, and the hierarchy is an arrangement that ranks the concepts from lowest to highest. To achieve success, the person must meet the needs at the lower levels before he or she tackles the next levels. The *Herzberg's Two-Factor Theory* states that there are certain factors in the workplace that contribute to job satisfaction and also a separate set of factors that lead to dissatisfaction. *Rogers' Change Theory* holds that innovations perceived by people that could have greater advantage for change should be adopted more rapidly than other innovations (Rundio & Wilson, 2010).

77. **D.**

Strategic planning is the development of an organizational strategy that will provide a long-term road map for a healthcare facility (Varkey & Bennet, 2010). *Succession planning* is part of strategic planning. *Contingency planning* the way the healthcare facility operates on a day-to-day basis, and it involves preparation for adverse events. *Program planning* is the organization's capacity to successfully execute a plan or service (Rundio & Wilson, 2010).

78. **B.**

Case study research involves investigation of a single individual or a group with similar diagnoses. Applied research is designed to solve a practical problem or answer a question. Descriptive research reports selected variables and proves facts that already are accepted. Experimental research randomly assigns participants with manipulation of variables (Rundio & Wilson, 2010).

79. **A.**

Field research is conducted in the natural setting. Historical research explains or interprets something in the past. Laboratory research is conducted in a setting designed for research. Longitudinal research involves measuring the same participants as they grow older (Rundio & Wilson, 2010).

80. **C.**

The *institutional review boards* (IRBs) exist to ensure that research participants are protected from unscrupulous and unethical practices and researchers. Guidance documents are posted on the FDA website and these guidelines represent the agency's current thinking on protection of human subjects in research (U.S. Food and Drug Administration, 2013). The National Advisory Council for Nursing Research (NACNR) provides second level review of grant applications and recommends which applications should be approved or considered for funding. *Nursing research councils* educate nurses about the importance of using research in clinical practice (National Institute of Nursing Research, 2013).

81. **B.**

Data is either qualitative or quantitative. *Qualitative data* involves the use of words to describe concepts, facts, participants' statements, and subjective observations. *Quantitative data* involves the use of numbers to enhance study precision. Three categories of quantitative data are: nominal data, which cannot be arranged in any particular order, such as marital status, religion, and race; ordinal data, which are ordered, but differences cannot be determined, such as socioeconomic status, car size, and facility ratings; and interval data, which are ordered and have meaningful differences, such as ratio data where there is an absolute zero (Rundio & Wilson, 2010).

82. **B.**

Validity means that the data-gathering instrument measures exactly what it is meant to measure. *Reliability* is how well or how consistent an instrument is for the purpose of a particular study. While an instrument may be able to measure something time and time again(reliable) without being appropriate (valid), an instrument may not be valid unless it is both reliable and valid (Rundio & Wilson, 2010).

83. **B.**

The eight dimensions of strategic innovation are: the managed innovation process, which combines non-traditional and traditional approaches to business strategy:

strategic alignment, which acquires internal support, industry foresight, which helps understand emerging trends; patient insight, which helps understand articulated and articulated patient needs; core technologies and competencies, which involves leveraging corporate assets; organizational readiness, which involves the ability to take action; disciplined Implementation, which requires inspiration to business impact; and sustainable innovation, which is a platform for ongoing competitive advantage (Strategic Innovation Techniques, 2002).

84. **C.**

The *divergence phase* is at the center of strategic innovation and is characterized as exploratory, open-ended, and creative thinking, which uses future visioning techniques. The *convergence phase* involves more traditional business development and planning, where potential opportunities are evaluated, selected, refined, and executed. There is no emergence phase (Strategic Innovation Techniques, 2002).

85. **E.**

The Equal Employment Opportunity Commission (EEOC) enforces equal employment laws involve various aspects of discrimination due to color, race, religion, age, national origin, sex, pregnancy, sexual orientation, and sexual harassment (U.S. Equal Employment Opportunity Commission, 2013a).

86. **D.**

With the Workers' Compensation law, an employee who becomes ill, or is injured on the job or from a condition caused by the worksite, is compensated for that incident. Workers' compensation is absolute liability for medical coverage, costs of rehabilitation, a percentage of wages or salary, and payment for permanent injury (not minor injury) (Rundio & Wilson, 2010).

87. **C.**

Collective bargaining is an agreement negotiated between an employer and a labor union that sets forth the terms of employment for workers who are members of that labor union. The term "collective" shows that agreements cover a defined population within an organization and are not individualized. A *grievance* is any complaint made by the involved parties. *Arbitration* is a process where a final and binding award is given by an arbitrator. A *contract* is a legally qualified agreement for a particular benefit of two or more people, which is a voluntary act (Rundio & Wilson, 2010).

88. **D.**

A *contract* is a legally qualified agreement for a particular benefit of two or more people, which is a voluntary act. Many states accept verbal contracts as legal contracts under this concept (Rundio & Wilson, 2010).

89. **B.**

Lateral thinking (also called innovative thinking) creates the idea, while vertical thinking (also called logical thinking) moves the idea forward. Critical thinking is the ability to analyzed a situation and use past knowledge to make decisions that are sound and fact-based (Mind Tools, LTD., 2013; Rundio & Wilson, 2010).

90. **D.**

The fee for service payment method involves a set price for a service. With healthcare, the amount paid for services is often negotiated between the provider and the payer. Under a *pay for performance* (PFP) approach, the healthcare insurer or other payer compensates healthcare facilities and physicians based on performance. The *pay for coordination* (PFC) payment applies to specified care coordination services by certain types of providers, such as home healthcare. With the *bundled payment* method, a single, bundled payment covers the services delivered by two or more providers during a single care episode over a certain period of time (American Medical Association, 2013).

91. **A.**

The hours per patient day (HPPD) is the total hours of nursing care that must be provided per patient per day. This value is determined by dividing total production hours by the number of patients (Rundio & Wilson, 2010).

92. **B.**

Part of the capital budgeting process is *amortization*, an assignment of costs to a capital item for its lifetime. This considers critically important aspects of the "life expectancy" of an item, which allows room for development of a replacement strategy. An operating budget, where revenue and expense segments are separated, allows for easy calculation of profit or loss. The *average daily census* measures inpatient volume based on the number of occupied beds or number of patients (Rundio & Wilson, 2010).

93. **B.**

Healthy People provides Americans with science-based, 10-year national objectives for improving health of all age groups. Healthy People 2020 reflects input from a diverse group of individuals and organizations and is a 10-year agenda for improving the nation's health. Objectives include increased public awareness of the determinants of health, disability, and disease, provision of objectives and goals that are applicable at the local, state, and national levels, and identification of critical research, data collection, and evaluation needs (U.S. Department of Health and Human Services, 2013a).

94. **D.**

According to the Agency for Healthcare Research and Quality (2013c), numerous health disparities were found in a recent report. These include: Blacks, American Indians, Asians, Native Alaskans, and Hispanics received worse care than Whites; poor or low income people received worse care than high income individuals;

Blacks, Asians, Hispanics, Native Americans, and Native Alaskans all had worse access to care than Whites; poor people had worse access to care than high income people; in 2005, Americans did not receive one third of the healthcare services needed; and in 2002, 24 percent of Americans had difficulties accessing health care, and by 2009, this had increased to 26 percent.

95. **D.**

The Affordable Care Act called for the creation of the Patient-Centered Outcomes Research Institute, which studies comparative effectiveness research that is funded by a fee on those insured. It also allows the FDA to approve generic drugs, with 12 years of exclusive use for new biologic medications. Additionally, this law involves programs that increase incentives to provide collaborative and quality healthcare (U.S. Department of Health and Human Services, 2013c).

96. **B.**

The Whistleblower Protection Act of 1989 protects federal whistleblowers who work for the government and report misconduct of an organization or agency. Whistleblowers can file complaints that they believe constitute a violation of: a rule, regulation, or law; gross mismanagement; gross waste of funds; abuse of authority; or a substantial, specific danger to public safety and health (U.S. Securities and Exchange Commission, 2011). The Health Insurance Portability and Accountability Act (HIPPA) of 1996 is a law that involves the electronic exchange and protection of healthcare information and patient data (Rundio & Wilson, 2010). The Fair Labor Standards Act (FLSA) establishes minimum wage, record keeping, overtime pay, and young employment standards for full-time and part-time workers in the private sector and in local, state, and federal governments (U.S. Department of Labor, 2013). Under the Civil Rights Act, employers cannot discriminate against an employee based on factors not related to job qualifications, such as age, sexual preference, religion, race, sex, or national origin (U.S. Equal Employment Opportunity Commission, 2013b).

97. **B.**

The Centers for Medicare and Medicaid Services (CMS) partnered with the Agency for Healthcare Research and Quality (AHRQ) to develop HCAHPS. These two Department of Health and Human Service organizations developed an initiative to provide a standardized survey instrument and data collection methodology for measuring patients' perspectives on hospital care (Centers for Medicare and Medicaid Services, 2013b).

98. **D.**

In a *decentralized system*, direct communication occurs in all directions and without restriction. With a *centralized system*, communication requires that input and output is controlled through a central point. A *local area network* (LAN) is several personal computers linked together through a server, and it allows for communication among organization personnel. A *wide area network* (WAN) is a system that is made of many LANs, where connections are affected by specialized networking software (Rudio & Wilson, 2010).

99. **A.**

Nurse compact legislation is a growing trend that is endorsed in most states, and model legislative language exists for licensure recognition. The *nurse compact* implies that state agencies must give up certain measures of parochial control of practice within their regions (Rundio & Wilson, 2010).

Made in the USA
Lexington, KY
15 August 2015